I Love U
Our Journey Through Autism

Timothy M. Arnwine

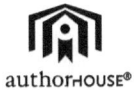

authorHOUSE®

AuthorHouse™
1663 Liberty Drive, Suite 200
Bloomington, IN 47403
www.authorhouse.com
Phone: 1-800-839-8640

First published by AuthorHouse 10/6/2008

ISBN: 978-1-4389-0717-8 (sc)

Library of Congress Control Number: 2008909021

Printed in the United States of America
Bloomington, Indiana

This book is printed on acid-free paper.

Dedication

This book is dedicated to our little man, Shane. He has completed our lives and allow us to celebrate the smallest victories that others take for granted.

To Shane's teachers, therapists, physicians, and other specialists who have touched our hearts.

To all the professionals who have chosen to work with children with autism, their devotion is greatly appreciated.

To all the parents of children with autism, their patience and unconditional love is to be admired.

Introduction

This book is not filled with scientific information, statistics, or medical jargon.

I am not a scientist, psychologist, or behavioralist. I am a former paramedic who specialized with children for many years. Presently, I am a stay at home dad and my wife Nancy, is a pediatrician. Although our education, training, and experience gave us some advantages, it could not prepare us for this devastating disorder. This is our journey through the challenges and victories of autism.

This book covers the time span from pre-birth, to give the reader a hint of our lifestyle to approximately Shane's fifth birthday. It shows a path from expected normalcy to the accepted reality of Shane's autism.

The goal is to show the reader that EARLY DIAGNOSIS, TREATMENT, AND THERAPIES ARE KEY TO THE BEST LONG TERM OUTLOOK FOR THE CHILD. I strongly suggest that you go with your instincts. Consult your pediatrician, a neurologist, or a psychologist. Become an advocate for the child as you would if you suspected any other medical condition.

From The Author

With early intervention, therapies, and great support from the autism community, Shane has made incredible progress, but compared to other families, we are fortunate.

Autism varies in severity, and there is a saying that illustrates this fact, " because you have met a child with autism doesn't mean you have met every child with autism".

As fortunate as we are, I never considered writing a book on this subject. I knew it would become an emotional roller coaster ride, having to relive the diagnosis and challenges. But one comment gave me a change of heart and a burning desire to take that ride.

I became involved with a fund raising walk for autism research. I called a physician friend who knows Shane to ask if he would sponsor me. He replied, I can not believe you are calling me for a donation, don't you know that autism is just another overused label, like A.D.D? I asked him, do your kids say I love you at bedtime? He replied, well yes. I responded, I know we would someday love to hear those same words.

As I hung up the phone, I realized that there is a great deal of ignorance to the facts of autism. Until recently, there has been little coverage and autism was kept in the dark shadows of our society. For most people, the only image of autism is the character from the movie, Rain Man.

Most children with autism have a normal appearance, therefore the parents must endure quiet whisperings about their parenting skills and impromptu medical advice from complete strangers.

I decided to write this book to help bring this devastating disorder out into the light.

This book is admittedly short, for two poignant reasons. One, as the parent of a child with autism, I know there is not much time to read. And more importantly, two, parents who suspect autism in their child do not have much time either, because early diagnosis and interventions are the key to your child's future.

This book gives the reader an insight into our lives to show that autism could and does occur in everyday families.

The goal is to give the reader a list to refer to as well as stories from our lives to better illustrate the signs of autism.

Contents

What Is Autism?
A Brief Overview

Autism is a brain disorder, causing deficits with communication and social skills. It is often associated with repetitive behavior, a lack of verbal skills, and difficulty accepting a change to their surroundings.

Autism affects 1 in every 150 children, which makes autism more frequent than pediatric diabetes, AIDS, and cancer combined. This disorder occurs in both genders, but more commonly in male children. Autism shows no prejudice, it occurs in all racial, ethic and socio-economical groups.

There is no known cause of autism or a cure. For Shane, early diagnosis was the key to gaining access to valuable interventions and therapies. Experts agree that early intervention can result in significant improvement of the child.

The following is a list of signs and other concerns of autism. The list was provided by Autism Speaks (www.autismspeaks.org). I would like to thank this wonderful organization for their tireless work with researching the cause and treatment for this devastating disorder.
Signs:

- Not babbled or cooed by one (1) year.
- Not gestured, pointed, or waved by one (1) year.
- Not spoke a single word by 16 months.

- Not spoke a two word phrase by two (2) years.
- Experiences any loss of any language skills at any age.

Other Concerns:

- Does not respond to his or her name.
- Cannot tell or describe what he or she wants.
- Experiences any delays.
- Does not follow directions at all.
- Appears at times to have a hearing impairment.
- Does not know how to play with toys.
- Has poor eye contact.
- Appears to be in his or her own world.
- Has odd movement patterns.
- Has unusual attachment to toys or other items.
- Regularly lines up toys or other items.

Initially, Nancy and I read a similar list. Taking the items one by one, we justified them as a minor delay or a typical two year old boy.

Experts agree that there is reason for concern if the child exhibits six or more of the impairments or any delays.

Chapter 1–
Our Life Before Shane

The Journey Begins

It was April 1, 1994 and I was working as a paramedic in the emergency room of a teaching hospital. A colleague told me that a pediatric resident was asking about me, initially I was apprehensive being that it was April Fools Day.

With curiosity and excitement, I had to meet this person. When I realized it was Nancy, I was thrilled. She is a beautiful Asian woman and was the sweetheart of the emergency room, everyone loved Nancy.

Shortly after that, we began dating and became inseparable. Since we did not drink alcohol, we were not the "clubbing types". We simply hung out together, went to movies, dinners and became best friends. We had a fun and loving courtship for five years. To this day, we still get teased about meeting on April Fools Day, since I have the reputation as the class clown.

From the start, I believed we would be married someday. We spent time together every day. After a three year engagement we decided to get married in December of 1999, while our friends and family were in town for the holidays.

Nancy was excited, not only about the vows but also the required shopping, a wedding dress. If shopping was in the Olympics, she would take the gold in both the marathon and dash. Nancy was so proud, she bought a beautiful wedding gown in ninety minutes. Spontaneity can be exciting, but someone must pay the price, I was the payee. It was December 26th and I took my daughter, Jessica into the lion pit of the local mall. After two hours of human bumper cars, feeling tired and bruised, we emerged into civilization with some wedding music for our big day.

The next day, Jessica and I decorated our house for a small ceremony. Afterwards, we had a post wedding dinner and toasted our new union with some bubbly apple cider. For the guys; present your wife with a pair of wedding date etched champagne glasses. It is both a gift and a way to always remember your exact wedding date.

We began our life as husband and wife. Nancy continued to work hard treating children in a private practice. We were able to do some things she missed out on. One, we attended every rock/pop concert and two, we started a family; of pets. Nancy was prevented from having a pet as a child, well…she caught up within two years. We started out with two rabbits, presently we have both dogs and cats to accompany the rabbits.

During my childhood, we had horses and always a house full of animals, both domestic and exotic, but I noticed something was missing in our house. We were missing that screaming kid chasing the pets and trying to stretch their tails.

The Decision

As the nursery rhyme goes, we had love and marriage, now comes the baby carriage.

For months, having a baby became more common in our daily conservations. I could give you the old stand by; we had so much love we had to share it, and that was a major reason. But I knew any child would be blessed to have Nancy for their mother and we wanted to give her parents a grand child.

Like anything else in life, there are obstacles to those things you truly desire. We had to consult an fertility specialist, I often joke with Nancy that I never seen a pediatrician get pregnant on their own. My theory is, because of the daily exposure to children screaming, the ovaries just say- there is no way that we are going to help create one of those.

I left the final decision up to Nancy, because I knew it would be a difficult road ahead. Nancy would have to endure injections, multiple blood draws and of course ; morning sickness and labor pains.

I am deeply grateful to her for making the sacrifice to bring Shane into our lives.

On a personal note, I respect any woman for the sacrifices they go through to have a baby, because if it was up to the guys, none of us would be here.

"Not Too Many Gloves"

As we began our research to find a fertility specialist, we spoke to many of our colleagues. We found an incredible physician in Ellen Wood, D.O. of The South Florida Institute of Reproductive Medicine.

Dr. Wood ordered blood tests as well as other specimen tests and we discussed our family history. Typically, both of our families are afflicted with the common medical conditions of high blood pressure, cardiac problems, and diabetes. Nancy could not recall any mental illness in her family. However, I remembered a cousin who passed on as a baby, I vaguely recalled he appeared to have some type of Down's Syndrome. There were also many gaps in our medical history due to the fact that my mother was adopted and Nancy's family is from Taiwan where information was not readily available.

After discussing our family history and considering our ages, I was closing in on forty and Nancy was thirty four years old. Dr. Wood suggested that we consult with a genetics specialist to rule any further complications.

After receiving the test results and the genetics report, Dr. Wood thought it would be safe to try and get pregnant. She then detailed our plan of action. As we discussed the plan, I began thinking ahead. I added up, a fertility specialist and the fact that my father is a twin, I suddenly had a vision of Nancy delivering a litter. I remembered pointing at Nancy's chest and saying you're going to have to grow six more breasts and lie down during feeding time.

Dr. Wood then gave me a baseball analogy, the idea is not to put up too many gloves to catch your guys. She was right, after two cycles of injections, Nancy was pregnant and according to the initial ultrasounds there was only one fetus.

I Love U

We Had a Baby... Seriously

Early into the pregnancy, Nancy had her days of nausea and exhaustion. The only complication was that Nancy developed gestational diabetes, which is a common pregnancy problem causing fluctuations in blood sugar levels. She was required to test her blood sugar daily and was prescribed medications to control her blood sugar levels.

As the pregnancy developed and Nancy's belly grew, so did our questions and doubts. Will the baby be healthy? Will we be good parents? There was one thing we did not doubt, who the baby would look like. Because in the gene pool, Asian genes rule the roost.

It seems we were always in a bookstore buying books on pregnancy and names. We read through internet articles, although we were medical professionals, we seeked the information to have a healthy pregnancy and delivery.

During the second trimester and after our reading, we agreed that Nancy should have an amniocentesis. An amniocentesis is a test for expecting mothers thirty-five years or older to detect possible abnormalities, such as Down's Syndrome or Spina Bifida. We also agreed, regardless of the results we would not abort the pregnancy. We simply wanted to know what lied in store. The results were negative for abnormalities and we were informed we were having a boy.

After discovering the sex, we began thinking of a name. We poured over the books and gathered suggestions from family and friends. We asked my daughter, Jessica for any suggestions. She suggested Mickey, after her favorite musical artist. I told her that I could not name him Mickey, because it gave me the image of that ill tempered trainer from the Rocky movies. But we agreed on Michael as a middle name and she could nickname him Mickey. After all the books and suggestions, it came down to a chance meeting for Nancy. She met a lady named

5

Shane, Nancy thought what a unique name and remembered the classic western movie character. So it was decided, we were waiting for the arrival of Shane Michael.

The next step in the natural order is how do we decorate the nursery. We decided to make blue bears the theme. Nancy, being the true shopping warrior and proud mommy to be, fought off exhaustion to go shopping; many times. By the time we were done, there were bear boarders and stuffed bears by the dozens and the crib was adorned with bear themed bedding. Nancy and I began collecting items for Shane. Nancy started collecting lunch boxes with cartoon characters and I collected baseball memorabilia items.

As an afterthought, we needed a cute nickname for him. My nickname for Jessica is "Pooh", so we wanted a name with same theme. Even though there would be a sixteen year age gap between them, we wanted Jessica and Shane to be close and a big part of each other's lives. We decided that Shane, being a boy would probably be very active and should be nicknamed Tigger.

Coming down the stretch, I was more excited everyday, while Nancy just wanted to see her feet and sleep on her stomach. Nancy was the guest of honor at that final ritual, the baby shower. I found myself being the only Y in a room full of X's. I was content to sit back and add to my sympathy weight gain. Looking back as I watched the festivities, I remembered thinking that Nancy is still the person that everyone loves. And to this day, we are grateful for those same friendships and their support.

As the date of Shane's arrival grew closer, Nancy and I discussed the possibility of me becoming a stay at home dad. We agreed that it was important for one of us to be home with Shane and since Nancy is a pediatrician, the choice was simple. I knew how fortunate we were to have the ability to consider the option that most families would take advantage of, if it were possible. After considering the regrets for all the times I missed watching Jessica grow up, I decided to trade my hundreds of kids at the emergency room for one child at home.

I remember what would be the final ultrasound, it was the best picture we got for the memories book. Shane's face was front and centered on the ultrasound screen. I told Nancy, look at his eyes- you can already tell he is Asian.

A couple of weeks later, April 1st rolled around. For most, it was the day of gags and pranks. It was more than that for us, it was the ninth anniversary of the day we first met. We felt great, the pregnancy was going as planned with the expectant date in approximately five weeks. Little did we know, Shane was planning to give us the ultimate April Fool's surprise.

It was 5:00 a.m. and Nancy was up early, she was on call and had to do rounds at the hospital. Nancy woke me up, she looked tired and told me she was restless all night due to cramps. My first thought was possibly false labor until she mentioned her back pain. As I mentioned earlier, I was a paramedic and had my fair share of delivering babies and recognized back pain as a sign of true labor. Usually, I am slow to wake up, my body gets up but my brain hit's the snooze button. But after I heard the words, back pain I was wide awake! I suggested to Nancy that she was in labor. She replied, I have to go in because I am on call. Well, I said; I am going to sit in this chair and you call me when somebody else confirms our suspicions. By 8:00 a.m., Nancy called- I'm in labor and already dilated 5 centimeters!

I jumped in the car, by the time I arrived at the hospital, Nancy was in the birthing room with an I.V. and attached to a fetal monitor. She appeared to be both nervous and surprised and I knew she had a story to tell.

She told me that during rounds, her cramps became more frequent and the back pain increased. Fortunately, our O.B. physician, Dr. H was also doing rounds and quickly responded to the hospital's page. Nancy met Dr. H on the labor floor and during the exam, her water broke. Dr. H knew it was time, but to everyone's surprise, Nancy asked if she could at least finish her rounds.

During the delivery, the only complication was to get Nancy to focus and push. Between the drugs and nervousness, Nancy was a chatterbox. But I know if that was me, I would be screaming. The delivery seemed to last forever, but shortly after 12:00 p.m.- Shane Michael arrived.

We asked the typical questions, does he have all his fingers and toes? Does he look healthy?

The only complication, besides being five weeks premature was that Shane had rapid breathing and would have to spend some time in the Newborn Intensive Care Unit (N.I.C.U.). I kissed and thanked Nancy for giving us a wonderful gift and let her get some well deserved rest.

As Nancy slept, I went home to care for our menagerie. I also made the phone calls to announce Shane's arrival. The first and easiest call was to Nancy's parents. Now, I am not sure if it was because of April's Fool's Day or that these people simply know me, but the rest of the calls were full of questions and doubts. After telling them the good news, first there was a giggle and then they would say; when Nancy is through having the baby- have her call us. I could actually feel the mid-air quote finger signs through the phone. I did receive one call back, my father phoned from Tennessee to ask if I was serious, because he was hitting the road to come see his new grandson.

As I drove back to the hospital, I was the one with a story to tell. As I walked into Nancy's room, I was embarrassed to tell Nancy that no one believed me and she would have to make the confirmation calls.

The phone calls would have to wait, because it was feeding time for Shane. As Nancy breast fed, we noticed he was a slow feeder. I remembered Shane met the criteria for jaundice. He was a premie, Asian, and a slow feeder, so we urged him to turn yellow so we could soon go home. Apparently, he understood us. By the next morning his breathing stabilized, but we had a day glow baby.

Shane spent the next two days in the N.I.C.U. on a bili blanket, which is the preferred treatment to control and reduce jaundice in newborns. While Nancy spent the final evening with Shane in the hospital, my father arrived. After a visit, my father and I went home to put the finishing touches on Shane's homecoming. I placed a large homemade birth announcement sign in the front yard and again there was doubt and questions. The morning we brought Shane home, the neighbors came to congratulate us and admitted they were somewhat skeptical if our sign was for real. Once the excitement subsided, we settled into our new life of diapers and two hour feedings.

Prelude to Stories

All major events in history have ended up with initials or a catch phrase for quick reference. When I mention B.C., WW II, or 9/11, everybody knows what I am referring to. When your child is diagnosed with autism, it may not be earth shattering news to the world but I guarantee it will be to you. Therefore, I have included P.D. (prior to diagnosis) and A.D. (after the diagnosis) in the title of the next two chapters to encompass certain age ranges.

The P.D. chapter refers to 0-2 years old. The A.D. chapter refers to 2-5 years old. Both chapters are comprised of stories in our daily lives. The A.D. chapter will also discuss the therapies and treatments we sought and took advantage of and their effects on Shane.

An Important Reminder

The following two chapters discuss the signs we observed and the concerns we had with Shane.

I believe and the experts concur, that early diagnosis is the key to have the best possible long term outlook for the child. Therefore, I have re-listed the signs and other concerns to be aware of as provided by Autism Speaks (www.autismspeaks.org). Separately, the items listed below could appear in most typical children. According to the experts, if a child exhibits six or more of these impairments, there is reason for concern. Before each story, I have noted the signs or concerns to look for and have placed Shane's signs in **bold** as they pertain to the list.

SIGNS:

    ( ) Not babbled or cooed by one (1) year.

    ( ) Not gestured, pointed, or wave by one (1) year.

    ( ) Not spoken a single word by 16 months.

    ( ) Not spoken a two word phrase by two (2) years.

    ( ) Experiences any loss of any language at any age.

OTHER CONCERNS:

    ( ) Does not respond to his or her name.

    ( ) Can not tell or describe what he or she wants.

    ( ) Experiences any delays.

    ( ) Does not follow directions at all.

(   ) Appears at times to have a hearing impairment.

(   ) Does not know how to appropriately play with toys.

(   ) Has poor eye contact.

(   ) Appears to be in his or her own world.

(   ) Has odd movement patterns.

(   ) Has unusual attachment to toys or other objects.

(   ) Regularly lines up toys or other items.

Through our experiences we were informed that other concerns were a factor in Shane's diagnosis.

(   ) Repetitive behavior.

(   ) Does not adjust well to a change in surroundings or routines.

(   ) Walking on "tippy" toes.

(   ) Increased level of pain tolerance.

(   ) Sensitive to touching different textures.

Within the stories, I use the term "meltdown". A meltdown is a tantrum that the child has, usually for no obvious reason. It is a confusing moment, because the parent has no idea of brought it on, therefore no way of calming the child or knowing what would prevent the next meltdown. In public, meltdowns usually bring on the "quiet whisperings" from strangers as mentioned earlier in the "From the Author" section. From my experience, each autistic child has their own twist on meltdowns. Shane's meltdowns would start with a scream and either he would either run to a "quiet' corner or thrash on the floor. This could be the tantrum of any child, it is part two, which I call the "re-focus period" that makes the difference. Shane would suddenly become silent and place his interlocked hands behind his head and stare for five or ten minutes. I have learned the hard way, that by rushing this re-focus period would only set off another meltdown which in turn becomes a viscous cycle.

Chapter 2 –
A New Journey—
Joy and Questions (P.D.)

The first few weeks, Nancy was home and we began to experience the normal cycle of sleep deprivation. Shane was still in the bili blanket at home for the first week. Between the diapers and the two hour feedings, we also experienced the two volumes of a newborn; quiet and screaming. Nancy, who is usually very active, was amazingly eager to relax and enjoy Shane. During this time, we greeted and proudly showed off our little man. The grandparents were frequent visitors. During these visits I created myself a schedule for household chores and childcare. I knew Nancy would soon return to work and it was my top priority to get this right. But soon reality took over and my schedule was gone, Shane was making the schedule.

The first few months were wonderful, but looking back I remembered there were subtle signs.

During the days, I found myself working around Shane's sleeping schedule because I did not want to miss a moment. As the weeks and months passed, Nancy and I began to notice some quirks in his movements and expressions. As medical professionals, our main concern was Shane's **periodic gazing/staring episodes**, because there is a medical condition referred to as petite mal seizures. These are a form of seizures that resemble "daydreaming". There were several situations where this gazing/staring was pronounced.

• No Babble/ Poor Eye Contact/Appears Hearing Impaired/ Not Responding to Name

From the first day we brought Shane home, our world revolved around him. Soon we were on the floor saying things like 'goo-goo, gah-gah" and 'gotcha' in that high pitched voice that all new parents develop. As the months passed, we graduated up to showing him items like balls and stuffed toys, saying his name and hoping for a response. For instance, I would hold up a bright multi-colored ball and Shane would **sit silently, turning his head away.** Even when I would physically guide his head towards the ball, **his eyes would deviate away and there was no verbal response**. By eighteen months, our hopes were turning to concerns. **Shane still had three settings- silence, screaming and the periodic belly laugh. There was no babbling or words**, like most parents we assumed he would be a late talker. Being naïve about his speech delay, we would simply make comments like, one day he will open his mouth and never shut up. I also teased Nancy by saying, hopefully he will be delayed long enough to get through the "NO" and "WHY" stage.

Any delay of speech should raise a red flag for possible hearing deficits. From three months old, **we noticed Shane would not respond to his name or any other noises.** I would tell Nancy that he was practicing to be a husband. These periods, although not constant would occur throughout the day, but differed from the staring episodes. It was obvious that he was enjoying his toy or activity, **because he would have busy hands and a stern focus. In order to get his attention,** we would have to grasp his face and bring it in line with ours, or during meal times we would gently tap his mouth with the spoon. After a few moments, we would have his attention, but still lacked the eye contact.

- In His Own World/Appears Hearing Impaired

During feedings, we were usually chasing his head up, down, and around, I would turn to get more food- turn back and realize he was staring into space. Our attempts to get attention by calling his name or tapping on the table always seemed to be on his terms. These episodes only lasted for a few moments and he would snap out of it with no obvious ill effects.

- Repetitive Behavior/ In His Own World

At approximately eight months old, he became obsessed with a new toy, that I call the ball/ramp toy. This toy came with four colored balls that you place through a hole to roll down a series of three enclosed ramps. With the balls constantly rolling, it was quite a noise maker. I remember thinking that Shane was easy to watch, as long as the balls were rolling, I knew he was safe. Shane would sit and roll the balls, usually for thirty minutes or more at a time. Periodically, the balls would stop prior to his usual thirty minutes, and when I checked on him, he was staring down towards the floor. Again, these episodes were short lived.

- Poor Eye Contact/ Does Not Know How to Play with Toys/ In His Own World

Between naps, we spent most of our time playing peek-a-boo or "gotcha" either in bed or on the floor. I also loved raising him above my head and do the baby talk. I recall when **I looked for a response, he would always turn his head away.** Even in those rare moments **when his head faced me, his eyes would deviate away.**

We had our daily parade of the stuffed animals but Shane **always seemed a thousand miles away**, and we noticed that he **never bonded with a stuffed animal.**

As mentioned earlier, we have a collection of pets and they have always been lovable towards Shane. The dogs loved sniffing and licking him, and the cats would rub up against him. There always seemed to be a **long delay until Shane responded to the animals.**

Personal Note:

Initially Nancy and I received a lot of advice to get rid of the animals. But I believe a well tempered pet can teach children to be gentle at their own pace. Fortunately, all of our pets have been patience with Shane. As he grew and became aware of the pets, he would not pet the dogs, he would pound them. I always had to remind him there is a reason they are called pets; not pounds and would show him the petting motion.

- No Changes in Surroundings or Routines/ In His Own World

I remember driving with Jessica as a child, the only problem was the constant- are we there yet? For a few months driving with Shane was pleasant, occasionally I had to look around to see if he was still there, I always found him **quietly staring out the window.** Then one day the silence broke! **While slowing for a red light, the Shane alarm began to blare.** I almost rear ended a car, looking back to check on him. **He**

continued to scream and thrash until the light turned green and we were moving. It was so common, that for sanity's sake, I would began to slow four to five car lengths behind the car ahead of us in traffic and inch up until the light turned green. I thought the scream/ no scream was better than the constant howling.

As new parents, time was a valued commodity and "drive thrus" became a dietary staple. Between Shane's meltdowns and the infamous restaurant speakers, I am surprised we ever got an order correct. The stopping meltdowns improved, but then we had a new challenge. **As soon as the person stuck their head out the window, Shane would begin to howl until we drove away then suddenly there was silence**. Eventually, we could only surmise that Shane thought the person was invading his space, even though they were outside of the vehicle.

- Ultra sensitive-Touch/ Nothing on Head or Neck/ Repetitive Behavior

As were the days, our nights were another learning experience. The nightly rituals of feedings and bathing became both stressful and confusing.

During feedings, we rarely hit the moving target; Shane's mouth. **We noticed that if he wiped his face or accidentally touched his food, he would frantically flap his hands** until we cleaned them. For us, this was confusing because **no matter the amount of food he touched, he always had "flapping episodes"**. Although, he did not seem to mind the food on his belly, legs or in his lap.

In the natural order, a bath was required. Feedings were a one man job, but a bath; especially hair washing had to be a team effort. Shane would tolerate his baths, **usually while lining up his toys or cups**. Washing his hair always required a strategy, for **as soon as the first**

drop of water hit his head, Shane began thrashing. While Nancy washed his hair, it was my job to keep him above water. After a quick towel dry, he would sit quietly by the tub and cover his eyes for a refocus period. We tried several "tear free" shampoo products to prevent the next meltdown. But finally, we surmised it was his reaction to the water on his head.

• No Changes in Routines or Surroundings

As Shane grew older, we decided to check our nerves and take him to restaurants . We loaded up on snacks to keep him busy. Initially it worked until the **server came to table, then Shane would have a meltdown**. He would either thrash or try to jump out of the high chair. I always took him outside, usually thrashing in my arms for a refocus period. After five or ten minutes I would try to bring Shane back into the restaurant but he always refused. We tried an experiment, I took Shane into fast food restaurants where there are no servers and he tolerated the experience longer each time. We slowly worked on our theory with slow diners and short stays at restaurants. After six or eight months, Shane grew accustomed to eating out, but periodically still has a meltdown. **Although to this day, Shane refuses to go into certain places if it is too dark or loud.**

• Nothing on His Head or Neck/ No Changes in Routines or Surroundings

Our first Halloween rolled around and we were very excited. Our neighborhood is very active, everybody decorates their house and we average fifty trick or treaters. We thought Shane would look cute as a dragon, he was adorable, but we had one problem, **he refused to wear**

the head piece. After his meltdown and refocus period, we were off the show Shane the decorations. **We got one house away, then Shane began flapping and pulling us back towards our house**. For the remainder of the evening, **each time the door bell rang, Shane would run to his quiet corner and crouched down**.

The Halloween horror night could have possibly been avoided if we thought it through. For months proceeding Halloween, we discovered that **Shane had a strong dislike for shirt tags**. He would **constantly grab at the nape of his neck or attempt to take his shirt off**. It quickly got to the point where all his clothes were washed in cold water, because we had to remove the tags including the washing instructions. This dilemma made buying his clothes difficult, we had to shop for return policies as well.

- No Changes in Routines or Surroundings/ In His Own World/ Lines Up Toys

The holidays are exciting, especially for new parents. We have always decorated both inside and outside the house. But this year the decorating duties were ten folded, if there was anywhere to hang or hook a decoration, it was used. Our house was a sampling of whatever was available for holiday decorations. As we decorated, we were excited for Shane, but became confused and disappointed when **Shane did not acknowledge all the beautiful lights and colors**. He would **simply sit by the tree lining up cups**. He periodically looked up as the cats climbed up the tree. Again our excitement grew as Christmas arrived. We spent Christmas Eve digging out the wrapped gifts from closets, the garage, and other hiding places. Without thinking, we placed a number of gifts where Shane would **usually sit to line up his cups**. Christmas morning, we were up early after a restless night of excitement of Shane's first Christmas. While Nancy woke Shane, I loaded the camera and video recorder to catch those first moments that each parent treasure. As he walked into the living room we were pleased to see him notice something new and for a fleeting moment we thought we hit the jack pot. **Instead of a wide eyed child, we had a screaming child running away from the area.** In retrospect, I believe **the meltdown occurred because the gifts were placed where he was accustomed to sitting**.

• Odd Movements/ No Pointing/ No Clapping

Finally, at approximately ten months old, he came to know the gang on Sesame Street, especially Elmo.

But with the glance of normalcy, we also recognized some new twists. I remember how pleased we were that Shane would actually sit still and by judging his expressions seem to enjoy watching Elmo. During this time we began to notice Shane would **smile and laugh but never clapped, instead he would have episodes of a hand washing motion or if standing, he would begin to spin around**. Once we noticed these impairments, we saw them in his everyday activities.

We were excited that Shane showed some interests in the Elmo toys we bought him. To promote this, we were constantly asking him if he wanted a toy. We then discovered that Shane would only respond to a particular toy, if we pointed it out. He **never pointed, he would simply hold out a hand when we touched the desired toy**. I am not sure if that is because these toys actually peaked his interests or were we "spoon feeding" him in those situations; probably the later.

• Repetitive Behavior/ In His own World/ No Changes in Surroundings or Routines

A first birthday is very exciting for the entire family. We planned a small family party at Nancy's parents. Nancy ordered special decorations, and when we arrived, the house had the appearance of a grand Sesame Street festival. For a brief moment, Shane recognized Elmo but **quickly sat down to play with his cups**. After a quick lunch, it was time for the cake and our tone deaf singing. Initially Shane was calm in his high chair and appeared to recognized Elmo again on the cake. Then as we **lit the candle and began to sing, he suddenly began to rock in the chair and had a meltdown**. I gathered Shane out of the chair to comfort him, but he just wanted to get down to go to a quiet corner. During his refocus period, we broke out the gifts, thinking new toys would cheer him up. As **we placed the gifts on the floor near him, he eventually noticed but quickly turned away screaming and thrashing**. As we drove home, I believe we had both confused and guilty feelings stirring. We were confused about the meltdowns and guilty about how we made Shane's first birthday such a traumatic event.

• Nothing on his Head or Neck

We approached all daily events as a team, from moral support to the periodic events where brute strength is required; like haircuts.

Shane was approximately one year old and had a beautiful head of hair, including a long set of ringlets. We began receiving compliments on our DAUGHTER. We even received some advice from a pleasant older gentleman of the Jewish faith. While trying to play with Shane, he pointed at his ringlets and said, "you know you can't cut these for three years".

We loved his hair but the combination of the comments and Shane's constant sweating caused us to get his first haircut. We took him to a place that specialized in children's haircuts. We thought the kiddie videos, colors, and cartoon characters would be a pleasant atmosphere. I placed him in my lap and for a moment, he was calm. Once again, we had no foresight. As soon as the lady **placed the smock around his neck, he had a meltdown**. Fortunately, the store was not busy, so we had time for a refocus period. After a few minutes I placed Shane on my lap again, only this time he was physically nervous, rocking and arching his back. This time with no smock, we were hopeful, but once the lady **sprayed his hair with water, he had another meltdown**, but being determined to get this done, we held on. Nancy held his head and I was in charge of legs and arms. Between the sweat and tears; including ours, it was like trying to keep down a greased pig. After fifteen exhaustive and stressful minutes we were done with what appeared to be a torture session. After Shane's refocus period, we gathered Shane off the floor to go home. We were both mentally and physically drained. After some thought, we should have remembered his hair washing episodes and considered the possibilities.

• Repetitive Behavior/ In His Own World

Our days together were wonderful, and I treasured every moment in Shane's world. But at eighteen months, we thought he would enjoy being around other children. We enrolled in a mommy and me, or in my case a Mr. Mommy and me class. It was so exciting to watch Shane jump and play in a new atmosphere. He enjoyed climbing, jumping, and playing with the balls, but **did not interact with the other children**. Very often, **I found myself sitting alone with the other mommies and children in circle time, attempting to coax Shane over from a ball and his solitude**. I always left the class beaming with pride, I was so pleased that he was trying new activities. After a few classes and my boastful stories, Nancy was eager to share in this small victory. Soon after that, Nancy was able to attend a birthday party. As we watched, I could sense she shared in my excitement, but then she asked a question that shined some light through my foggy pride. She said, does he always do the same thing? Then I realized, **he always followed the same pattern of climbing and jumping on the play equipment and would briefly participate in circle time for the parachute game**. After that, the next few classes became somewhat stressful as I tried forcing Shane into participating in circle time, which resulted in numerous meltdowns and refocus periods. Until his diagnosis, we kept him in the class for the sole purpose of allowing him to enjoy himself. After the diagnosis, we decided that Shane should be in a more structured atmosphere.

Chapter 3 –
Our Journey into the
Black Hole (A.D.)

Shortly before Shane's second birthday, our concerns pushed us to get some answers on delayed speech.

We took advantage of Shane's sleep over at his grandparents to go to the local bookstore to do some research on the subject. While I was reading through delayed speech and sign language books, Nancy picked up a book on autism. While flipping through the pages, we found a list of sixteen items and suddenly our concerns turned into fears. As we read through the list, we tried to reason away each item. But one line felt like it jumped off the page and kicked us in the gut. IF THE CHILD EXHIBITS 6 OR MORE OF THESE IMPAIRMENTS, THERE IS REASON FOR CONCERN. Shane exhibited 15 of the 16 impairments.

To use an old cliché, timing is everything. The reason Shane was staying at his grandparents was that Nancy and I had tickets for a rock concert, which we were excited about attending. Our research and the thought of the possibilities numbed our enthusiasm, but we decided to go as a diversion. As we sat there trying to recapture a portion of our past, I sobbed; thinking about our little man and his future. Nancy was obviously upset, but was determined to stay strong until we got a confirmation of our fears. Then fate took a hand into our lives for a brief moment. On Sunday morning, the day after the concert I went to the local mall just to get out of house. I ran into two members of the band, we had coffee and talked about classic rock bands. As I left, I told them about my admiration for their music and thanked them for the concert as it was a great diversion for us. I then relayed our story of Shane possibly being autistic, and the lead singer told me that he has two nephews with autism, they are now teens and have really improved over the years. I left there with the feeling of a better future.

Within a week we had an appointment with Dr. Tucchman, a well respected neurologist who specializes with autistic children. Initially, Dr. Tucchman observed Shane and attempted to get his attention, but to no avail. Then he pulled out the same type of ball/ramp toy that Shane had at home, and suddenly he had Shane's attention. I remember saying to Dr. Tucchman, you have made a friend, he plays with that toy all the time. Moments later, he said I don't think so. I think we have got a problem, then he confirmed our fears, that Shane was autistic and explained the spectrum of severities.

After the diagnosis, it took approximately a week for the news to settle in that our lives have changed. During that time I kept telling Nancy, I just want him to be happy. From that moment on, I found myself pretty open about Shane's diagnosis to family, friends, and even complete strangers if the situation presented itself. For me, it was therapeutic, the more I said it the more it sunk in. The fact is, Shane is autistic and we just have to face it and find ways to help him.

Since I was so open with Shane's diagnosis, I was commonly asked, how did he get autism? Honestly, we never spent much time or energy on the cause, we focused on treatments and therapies. I have become active in Shane's school and learning his rights to become the most affective advocate for him, which I feel is my most important role to support him.

High Pain Tolerance

A high tolerance for pain is not included in the opening list of signs and other concerns. I have included this section due to the fact that most parents of children with autism that I know, agree their children also have a high tolerance for pain. I believe this should be a medical concern that each parent of a child with autism should be aware of.

- High Tolerance for Pain/ Odd Movements/ Ultra Sensitive Touch

For infants, their first predictable cause of pain is usually their shots.

At three weeks old, Shane began his regiment of vaccinations. Initially, Shane would have the normal delayed reaction to pain that we have seen in other children. But at approximately eighteen months old, we began to notice **he would feel the need to sit quietly on the floor with a hand washing motion after his shots**. At two years old, we were made aware that he was unable to verbally express a reaction to pain.

As Shane grew older, he experienced the normal bouts of colds and ear infections, but now he required "finger sticks" for blood tests. During these tests, we were truly made aware of his high tolerance for pain. We were **amazed that he would sit quietly and look down during the actual "finger stick", but would have a meltdown while we attempted to apply a gauze or band-aid to his finger**.

Shane may be autistic, but he is all boy; he runs, climbs, and has had his share of bumps and bruises. We have gone to great lengths to child proof our home, but we have had a few experiences where Shane has walked up rubbing his bloody nose or his head. We usually, ended up rubbing our heads wondering what happened, because **he never cried out**.

Through our experiences, we have come to expect the unexpected. On a daily basis, we walk the fine line of watching over him, but not smothering him.

PERSONAL NOTE:

The word vaccine is now synonymous with autism. Through our research of medical journals and publications, we found the findings to be inconclusive for the cause of autism. As earlier suggested, follow your instincts. For us, we agreed that the long proven positives of vaccines outweigh the possible negatives. In the future, science may prove we made a horrible error in judgment, but as previously discussed, we do not dwell on the "what if's". We would rather focus on his therapies and daily structure. To date, Shane still receives his required vaccines and there have been no sustained signs of increasing delays or regressions.

Early Intervention= Strong Foundation

After Dr. Tucchman pulled back the curtain and confirmed our fears, he recommended the first person who would play a major role in Shane's life.

Within a week, we met Monica Ventura, a speech pathologist. Although Shane never interacted or even looked up, she showed the greatest patience and a sincere concern for our little man. Immediately, Nancy and I felt confident that she could definitely help him and agreed to two sessions per week.

Added to our cauldron of emotions was now excitement and apprehension. We were excited because we were starting his therapy and had a comfortable feeling about Monica. The apprehension came from the unknown, because we did not know what to expect or if he would even respond to speech therapy. As we left our first session, I felt more confident in our decision to work with Monica. I was able to sit on the first session and again was awed by her patience. I was pleasantly surprised to see that her teaching tools were toys; for two reasons. One, I knew she would use the concept of fun and play and two, I could learn some techniques and use the same toys at home to help with his therapy. Remembering the importance of structure, I was grateful when Monica agreed to show me the techniques and play style in order to duplicate his therapies at home.

Beginning with the second session, Monica thought it would be best to work alone with Shane. My stress level jumped, only because it was the first time I completely gave Shane to somebody else. Initially, I thought I would have to sneak a listen through the door, but I found that it was not necessary as I could hear him screaming into the lobby. The screaming tore out my heart and those thirty minutes seemed like thirty hours.

Over the next few sessions, Monica introduced us to a new toy. It was a barn shaped toy where Shane would place a coin like piece into a slot then push down a lever to retrieve the piece. The catch was that he first had to knock on the toy in order to push the lever. To my surprise, the purpose of this was to start developing a sign language so we could better communicate.

Monica made us realize that by leaving all his toys and snacks within reach, he would never grasp the basic skill of conveying his wants and needs. We began to place his snacks out of reach and toys in see through locked containers. We also began training Shane to point in order to teach him to give a specific sign for the desired container or snack. He also would have to knock on it as a way of asking for help. We incorporated this exercise into everyday basic needs, such as opening a door.

As we began his therapies, we felt the true frustration of being the parent of a child with autism. I believe that was the first time we realized the monumental task set before us and would be a life long journey.

As a rookie in this game, I was grateful for the simple explanation of autism. My understanding was that Shane's brain was wired differently. He would require a constant and repetitive flow of therapy, just to learn the basics.

Typical children usually learn to point as well as other basics from their peers, Shane had to learn by physically showing him the motion. I found myself literally prying his pointer finger from a clinched fist dozens of times a day. To this point, his meltdowns usually occurred due to something beyond our control, but now we were purposely changing a routine and dealing with constant meltdowns. After a few months, we scored a major victory when he independently pointed and knocked on a door he wanted to be opened. As I sat there crying, I felt elated for

Shane and sad for Nancy, because usually, at least one parent will miss a major event in their child's life, this was ours. For the next four to six months while constantly working on this exercise, he began to master pointing and knocking with few regressions; another victory. During this time, we worked on getting his attention and a sign to communicate that he has either grown tired or completed a task.

In order to get his attention, I had to physically grasp his head and while repeating his name I would touch my nose until he responded with some degree of focus.

Eventually, with some success we were able to create other signs like, get down or come here. The sign we created for a completed task was a hand swiping motion, a minor victory. Shane never physically initiated this, but gained a good understanding of the meaning and would positively respond to it.

After months of therapy, we began to see positive changes in Shane and felt confident that we would someday be able to have some form of communication. Suddenly, we had a major set back, we lost Monica as Shane's therapist.

During their time together, we began to experience a new emotion; hope. Even though Monica recommended her associate Erica Grub, whom we have met several times, once again we some apprehensions regarding his future. We were confident that his session routine would not change but pondered if there would be any regression during the adjustment time to a new therapist. I do not believe Erica and Shane ever achieved the same connection that he had with Monica, but Erica introduced us to another important system to aide in his development. The system is known as PECS (Picture Exchange Communication). PECS are a system used for non-verbal communication, where the child interacts using a visual representation of the desired task or object. Erica's use of PECS were incredible, she combined the picture of a desired object and our recorded voice, to serve both as a communication device and a teaching tool. For example, if Shane wanted a boxed juice, he would have to push the button on the picture frame and give a positive response (point) to the repeated question, do you want juice?

We remained with Erica for a few months until a conflict of schedule with Shane's Pre-K made it impossible.

We will always be grateful for their time in Shane's life. Today, thanks to these two special women we can now see how early intervention has built a strong foundation for Shane's future.

Cow Hunting

• Odd Movements

While working with Erica, we noticed that Shane was becoming more verbal. Up to this point, his vocabulary consisted of two garbled words; open and up, but only when prompted.

While driving around, we noticed he would periodically say "oooo". After a few confusing days, we realized that he would say "oooo" while driving by a cow pasture. It was then that we realized that "oooo" could be moo. It was another victory for Shane, it was the first time that he appropriately verbalized a sound with spontaneity. With excitement and an eagerness to build on it, we took daily drives by that same pasture and even traveled throughout South Florida to look for other pastures. After several trips to the pasture, we found the herd grazing by the fence. As I slowed to show him the cows, he began to kick with excitement and displayed his **hand washing motion**. After repeated "oooo's" I decided to take a chance and pull off the road. I wanted to allow him the chance to get up close and personal with these animals that obviously intrigued him. I enjoyed watching a picture from one of his books suddenly come to life in his eyes.

As I gathered him from the car, I felt that excitement turned to fear as he stiffened like a board and the **hand washing motion** turned to **hand flapping**. Shane began to loosen up the closer we got to the fence, he was silent with a look of fascination. Suddenly, he began with a series a "happy shrieks", which caused a slow stampede of the cows from the area.

Because of his fascination for all animals, we were able to build a form of sign language. We would use the sounds and features of the animal to create of type of matching game from his books. We have taken dozens of trips to zoo's, aquarium's, and other attractions where animals are on display. For us, this was an amazing time, we were finally a part of something that Shane would respond to.

Never Assume- Ask!- Ask!- Ask!

During our time with Erica, we were excited about Shane's progress. We began to believe that "more is better", but unfortunately Erica's schedule was full , so we searched for additional speech therapy. We found an organization that provided in-home therapy for children with autism. After an evaluation, we were delighted to hear that they agreed to send a therapist for two hour sessions, twice a week.

By now, we were not so naïve about his autism and realized this would be a difficult adjustment for him. One major adjustment would be the two hour sessions and another would be the new therapists.

The first few sessions were as expected, a string of meltdowns. During these meltdowns, the therapists showed incredible tenacity and patience with Shane. I was realistic and knew that if Shane was to grow, there would be rough times.

As I observed the sessions, I felt like something was not right. One, they were constantly referring to a three ring binder book. This gave me the impression that each situation was black and white with no variables for each child. The second observation was that their expectations were unrealistic for Shane's development. Even though Shane had no signs of spontaneous verbalization, they were requesting that he learn to speak ten syllables by the next session.

Fortunately, we had a follow up appointment with Dr. Tucchman prior to the next session. I relayed my concerns during Shane's exam and he suggested we discontinue the in-home therapy because they appeared to be Behavioral Therapists. After confirming his suspicions, I was surprised. My initial contact and evaluation was based on difficulty with speech, so naturally I assumed they would send Speech Therapists.

At this point, we were not aware of Behavioral Therapists. To be the best advocate for your child, do your research and ask questions.

Chapter 4 –
Life Goes On

We knew our lives have changed, but at the same time we realized that life goes on and we could not just shove Shane into a closet. There were errands to run and also fun outings to help stimulate him.

We anticipated the usual challenges of meltdowns and the whisperings of others, but it was our desire to give Shane a sense of normalcy. I was surprised with my patience and tolerance of others, although there were times when diplomacy had to take a back seat. Unfortunately, on some occasions I had to use the shock value approach to make my point.

• Refocus Period

Like most parents, I would take Shane to the mall for lunch and let him run off some energy. Once, I remember Shane had a meltdown and during his re-focus period, **Shane lied on the floor staring at the ceiling**. I heard some lady whispering-"why doesn't that dad do anything"? She finally walked over and asked, if I am going to let him just lie there? Sarcastically, I said- lady look at him; he is just catching rays and thinking about life. While she gave me a blank stare, I said,

I think more adults should take time to do the same, don't you agree? She quickly walked away, whispering other things.

- Tippy Toes Walking

As I mentioned before, Nancy and I work as a team. There have been occasions where I have handed Shane to her as she walked in from work. Although Nancy never asked, there have been many times where I have taken him out for a hour or two to give her some down time.

One of our favorite places to go is the baseball park, where he can run and climb on the bleachers. It is always uplifting to chase that little man and listen to his addictive belly laugh. One night while watching Shane, I forgot about our problems and got lost in the moment, when suddenly a voice snapped me back to reality. I looked up and there stood a young lady holding a beautiful baby. With a concerned look on her face, she kept repeating, **do you know he walks on his tippy toes**? Now, I have learned one thing through this experience. Every unsolicited piece of advice is followed by their opinion, comprised into one line- "I would have that checked out". For some reason, **Shane's tippy toes walking** became the focus of her life, or at least ten minutes of it. As we walked, this woman followed us, pointing out the obvious and making her opinion known, which I always retorted- we have had his walking checked out. Finally, after ten minutes, I felt the shock value approach was appropriate. I said, I appreciate your concern, but actually we want him to become a ballerina. He has the foot work down, but he is lacking the frontal bulge that other male ballet dancers have, with her mouth agape she suddenly disappeared from our lives.

- In His Own World/ Not Talking

Living in South Florida, we have our yearly bouts with hurricane threats, which usually results in long lines at the grocery store for supplies.

When Shane was two years old, we found ourselves in one of these lines. While he sat quietly in the cart, I was double checking our items determined not to return to this madhouse. I briefly looked up when I heard this lady repeatedly saying- hello, what is your name? I felt sorry for her, because I knew **he would never acknowledge her presence**. In retrospect, I should have mentioned his condition and thanked her for her effort, but instead I continued. Moments later, I felt a tap on my shoulder and she asked me, **doesn't he talk**? And I replied, **no-not yet**. As I continued to check our items and answer repeated inquiries about Shane, I noticed he began his rocking motion as she got closer to his face. I felt another shock value approach was required. Frustrated, I said, lady if he said #@*# off right now I would be the happiest guy on earth. Well, I guess she had time to kill because she moved to another (much longer) line.

There have been occasions where the reaction from strangers were smiles and compliments. Inside we experienced both happy and sad emotions. We were happy to see Shane enjoying himself, but sad because we knew he was usually in own world.

- Odd Movements/ In His Own World

As any other child, Shane was invited to many parties.

We once attended an outdoor party at a small quiet park. Admittedly, it was a child's party where the adults were friends and Shane had never met the other children. We were happy to hear his belly laugh as he ran around watching the other children in the bounce house. Then suddenly, he began pulling us towards the front of the bounce house, where to our surprise he apparently wanted to join the other children. Although he never actually joined the others, I remembered fighting back the tears while watching Shane jump and play like a typical boy. Time seemed to stop and we encouraged him to stay so we could enjoy another victory. But only moments later, he made his way to the front and signaled us to get him. As Nancy plucked him out, I was amazed. Because I did not see fear, I saw a smile and he showed a **hand washing motion**, which was Shane's sign of excitement.

As the party moved under the pavilion, I was holding him and catching up with old friends. As the noise level grew, Shane began to stir in my arms with a sudden urge to get down. With some excitement, I told Nancy- look, he wants to go back to the bounce house. But sadly enough, once again we misread his intentions. He proceeded to the center of the pavilion floor, **he covered his ears and spun around**. Although we knew the reason for this behavior, we gathered our inner strength to join the other parents as they smiled and enjoyed Shane's floor show. While watching him, I whispered to Nancy- look, he's having an "A" moment.

• Odd movements/ In His Own World/ Repetitive Behavior

Nancy and I are both baseball fans and fortunate to have a two time World Series championship team in our backyard. We are also fortunate to have access to tickets for several games during the season, thanks to Nancy's office.

Since the tickets were basically a gift and we look for new experiences for Shane, we thought we would test our nerves and take him with us. We were anxious to see how he would react to the crowd and noise.

We arrived early to ease him into this new atmosphere. While Nancy shopped for souvenirs, Shane and I watched the players warm up. As they hit and ran for the ball, he seemed excited with his beautiful smile and **his hand washing motion**. As the singing of the National Anthem neared, fearing that the noise would ruin this experience, I hurried him up to the concession area for refreshments. Although the noise was muffled, Shane **covered his ears and found a corner to crouch down**. After the singing and a re-focus period, he reluctantly agreed to go to back to our seats. As we made our way back, my only thought was, how long could he tolerate the actual game.

To our amazement, we were about to have another learning experience. We learned that Shane loved popcorn and zippers. After several attempts, he discovered the joy of popcorn and practically ate the entire bucket. As a habit, Nancy never carried a purse to outings like a ballgame, she would wear a fanny pack containing only five to six items. With Shane sitting between us, it was during the second or third inning when he **unzipped her pack and began to hand me each item one by one, he then returned them in the same order and re-zipped the pack**, and the marathon was on.

While we enjoyed the game, both on the field and in our seats, once again the quiet whisperings arose. This was an exception, the surrounding fans were complimentary. They were remarking on well he sat still and behaved. Before we knew it, it was the seventh inning and we decided to leave in order to beat traffic. As we left, we received numerous compliments and even a couple of " I wish my child was like yours at the ballgame". Internally, I believe we wanted to take credit for our parenting skills, but sadly enough we knew the reason for his behavior, so we returned a gracious smile and thank you.

Since then, there have been occasions where we have repeated the same magic and other occasions; complete meltdown. Perhaps the timing was off or a louder noise level. Yet, depending on the situation at home, we always attempt to take Shane to the ballgame whenever we have tickets.

• In His Own World/ Ultra-sensitive Touch

Living in South Florida, there is another gift from mother nature you can experience; the beach. We have never been beach goers, for me, sand just find its way into too many weird places.

I do not recall his exact age, but it was before the diagnosis. My father was visiting and we decided to take Shane to a beach boardwalk to introduce him to the ocean. While grandpa strolled him towards the boardwalk, I prepared the video camera to catch his first expression as he noticed the ocean. As we rolled him onto the boardwalk, we noticed **he was fixed on his stroller toys**. We spun him around, tried different angles and I even tried that useless term, TA-DA! Like I suddenly created the ocean. As I jumped and flapped my arms trying to get his attention, I had a humbling revelation. I realized you can be on a crowded boardwalk and the quiet whisperings could come from within. I believe that this was the first time I had real concern for Shane. **I was amazed that my antics, the passer-bys, the seagulls, and the ocean sounds could not divert his focus**.

A couple of years have passed and we had our diagnosis, and on a whim I thought we would try another beach outing.

As we arrived on the boardwalk, this was a different child and I was about to enjoy another small victory. He was flashing that beautiful smile and pulling me towards the water. As I laid down the towels, I noticed Shane was gazing at the waves. To my surprise, the waves and noise did not seem to bother him. After numerous attempts, he was standing in the surf! With great pride, I slowly led him further into the water. As we walked out of the water, a wave came up and knocked him down. I pulled him up to find a happy boy with a nervous laugh. After a hug, he went back into the surf and as he knelt to play, I felt a sense of normalcy in our little man. Moments later, he sprang up **flapping his hands and signaling for me to wipe his hands**. As I wiped his hands, I remembered his reaction to touching food as an infant. I realized he is probably hypersensitive to the feel of different textures as we were forewarned by his neurologist. We played for a few moments, repeating the process and he decided it was time to go home. While driving home, I was celebrating another victory and feeling the disappointment of a new obstacle.

Chapter 5 –
Just Tell Me He's Bad Enough....

As Shane's third birthday approached, we began to consider his education. We realized he would require a specialized curriculum with strict structure and that various therapists would have to be involved.

Although we were familiar with early therapies for which we had complete control, we were naïve about the educational system for children with autism.

Once again, we turned to our trusted allies in this fight, Shane's team of therapists and physicians. They informed us that we had the right to tour our local public school that provided pre-kindergarten services.

I made arrangements to meet the teacher, see the facilities and find out what they could offer our little man. I approached the tour with an open mind, and a long list of questions. The teacher was pleasant and appeared to be enthusiastic about working with special needs children. Throughout the tour, I remember that doubt began to close my mind to a few concerning remarks that were made, such as "we are planning on this" or " I want it to be like that". I began to think with only a few weeks before the start of school, this class was still in the planning stages.

As a parent of a child with autism, I believe I had one responsibility that must be focused on; to become his strongest advocate.

We knew we could not just settle for whatever was available, especially in the early education process. Frantically, we began to look for other options to discuss with the Broward County School's Psychologist during Shane's upcoming evaluation.

As we gathered advice from Shane's team and our colleagues, one school name kept popping up, The Baudhuin School.

Baudhuin is a pre-kindergarten school with an excellent reputation for their dedication and commitment to children with autism.

Our focus quickly changed to get Shane enrolled into Baudhuin. We thought, with his diagnosis and Dr. Tucchman's reputation, enrollment would be automatic.

Once again, our emotions were riding high, but about to take another hit. During the process, we learned that in order to get into Baudhuin, a licensed psychologist or psychiatrist (not a neurologist) must diagnose the child as autistic. With that one piece of information, our confidence sank, because we realized Shane's upcoming evaluation with the psychologist was so important to his future.

The eve of his evaluation was a restless night. As odd as it sounds, our main concern was, what if Shane goes to the evaluation and has a good day? Because we knew with the services that Baudhuin could offer, Shane could have a strong foundation.

The day of the evaluation, we met Sherry Swanson, who lead the evaluation team. During the evaluation, he did not miss a beat. He showed his repetitive behavior and although they were caring people and attentive to him, Shane never acknowledged their presence. After thirty minutes, the moment came, those four tragic words again; your son is autistic. This time I thought I was mentally prepared, but as Sherry gently leaned forward and with a soft voice to tell me what we already knew, my eyes welled up. As I composed myself and wiped away the tears, I responded, okay, but tell me, is he bad enough to get into Baudhuin? She gave me a look of total surprise, and I suddenly had sympathy for her. I remember thinking, how sad it must be for her, that quite often she is probably the first person to break the news to a family.

Although it was difficult to watch the evaluation and relive the diagnosis, we had another victory for Shane with his acceptance to Baudhuin.

"Hoping"

In today's world, we are inundated with hype. Hype about restaurants, products, and movies. I remember hearing numerous times from people who have seen a movie, " I wish I had those two hours of my life back". Well, two hours is a mere flicker in a child's life.

Hype is anything positive you hear from someone else. I guess we were excited and bought into the hype of Baudhuin. But we will always be grateful that everything we heard was true about Baudhuin.

The "Bubble"

Our first morning at Baudhuin was a humbling experience. For the first time, we were in a room with a large group of children with autism that covered the entire spectrum of severity. Everyday we woke up to the reality of Shane's autism and still had bouts with self pity. But this particular morning definitely changed our perception. Although we saw Shane in many of these children, some were severely autistic and I thought how fortunate we were and should just count our blessings.

It was refreshing to see that during a meltdown, there was no over reaction from the staff or rolling eyes from other parents. There was simply a gentle touch and words of reassurance from the staff and "veteran" parents. As I began to meet the other new parents, I saw the frustration in their eyes and the exhaustion on their faces. It was then that I realized that sadly, we were part of a unfortunate club. The membership dues were hefty, but the support and encouragement have been incredible.

I am not sure why, but there seem to be moments where you could simultaneously hear dozens of conversations. Some veteran parents were grateful for the break being over, while others were saddened that they were beginning their last year at Baudhuin, what they lovingly refer to as the "bubble".

As the door opened, I remember the knots in my stomach begin to loosen, because all the comments were positive from the parents who entrusted their children to the staff.

As we walked the hallway to his classroom. Shane quietly took everything in stride while we choked back the tears.

At his classroom, we were met by his teacher, Miss Nicole Gaskin. A soft spoken woman with an air of kindness. After stealing a hug from Shane and a comforting "he will be alright" from Miss Nicole, we left our little man in her hands. As we left the class, there was a degree of relief, because now we could cry.

The drive home was silent with the occasional sniffle as we absorbed this new chapter in our lives.

Our first morning without Shane allowed us a luxury we have missed, breakfast in restaurant without the fear of a meltdown. As we discussed our morning, I discovered that we shared the same torn feelings. We were happy there were no tears or screaming from him as we left. But selfishly, we were saddened by the absence of any separation anxiety that the typical child would have displayed.

Our time alone was pleasant but we were eager for two o'clock, when we could go get our little man. While walking into his classroom, we did not expect Shane to run into our arms screaming momma and dada. But strangely enough, we seemed to expect a response to questions about his first day. Once again, my heart sank as I turned around to see him staring blankly out the window. The first few weeks of school seemed to calm our nerves. Shane was adjusting to the changes and appeared to be happy. Even though we saw no changes, we had our minds set in realty and were not expecting a magic pill. Looking back, I believe that this time was more for us, the parents. We began to build bonds and look to each other for support. Through the veteran parents, we were learning about our children's teachers and aides. It was comforting to hear that every comment regarding Miss Nicole was positive and were told numerous times how fortunate we were to have her as Shane's teacher.

There was another major positive during this time. We met Manny Gonzalez-Abreu, Ph.D., known as Dr. Manny, the door man. We soon discovered that the gentleman who opened the door and greeted us each morning would become a great influence on us. He always made time to give advice or listen to our concerns. For us, Dr. Manny also opened our minds to all the possibilities for Shane. I strongly suggest that you find a "Dr. Manny" in your school or community to help ease your travel down this rocky path.

I have learned there are two important tools for the parents of a child with autism. You need support, but more importantly, you need the knowledge about your child's autism and their rights. At Baudhuin, Dr. Manny either led or organized the parental classes and support groups.

He introduced us to three letters, I.E.P.. Though we were not aware of the importance of this process, we saw the anxiety effect it had on parents going through it.

I.E.P. (Individual Educational Plan) is the cornerstone for the education of a child with a disability and individualized for that child's needs. The I.E.P. process may be termed differently in your area, check with your local school system.

The I.E.P. falls under I.D.E.A. (The Individuals with Disabilities Education Act- P.L. 101-476). This is an amended version of the Education for All Handicapped Children (P.L. 94-142, 1975). In 1997, I.D.E.A. was reauthorized (P.L. 105-17), which further defined the child's rights and strengthened the role of the parents in the process.

I.E.P. meetings must be held annually. If necessary, interim meetings can be requested. The school or agency must attempt to schedule a meeting that is agreeable to both school staff and the parents. By law (CFR 300.344), the following people must be invited:

- Parents/ Guardians
- Student's teacher
- A representative of the public agency, other than the teacher.
- The child, if appropriate.
- Other individuals at the discretion of the parents/ guardians (i.e.-physician, therapist, advocate, neighbor, etc.)

The I.E.P. should list the educational services to be provided and the professionals who will provide the service. The list includes:

1. Child's present level of educational performance.

- Strengths of the student
- Effect of the child's disability on their educational performance.
- Priority of needs.

2. Objective Criteria, evaluation procedures and schedules to determine if the child is achieving the short tem objectives

3. A statement of goals which the student may reasonably accomplish in the next 36 weeks, including a list of intermediate objectives for each goal. The areas that may be addressed include, but not limited to:

- Communication
- Behavior
- Socialization
- Sensory needs
- Academics

I.D.E.A. requires that goals must be related to meeting the child's needs that result from the disability.

4. Description of specific special education and *related services.

- Regular Educational Programs
- E.S.Y. (Extended School Year)
- * Related Services (Defined by I.D.E.A.) include and must be written into the I.E.P.
- Audiology
- Counseling

- Early Identification and Assessment
- Medical Services for Diagnostic or Evaluation Purposes
- Occupational Therapy (O.T.)
- Parent counseling and Training
- Physical Therapy (P.T.)
- Psychological Services
- Recreation
- Rehabilitation
- School Health Services
- Speech Pathology
- Transportation

IMPORTANT !!

I.D.E.A. establishes the minimum requirements schools must provide. The state may exceed the requirements and provide more services. They cannot provide less or have state regulations or practices that contradict the guidelines of I.D.E.A.. The state must provide an appropriate educational program for the needs of the child.

At the conclusion of the I.E.P. meeting, you must be provided with a copy at no cost to you. You will be asked to sign the I.E.P., however, this does not conclude that you are in agreement with the school or agency. It simply acknowledges that you were present at the meeting.

If you and the school/agency have a disagreement on the I.E.P., you can utilize one or more of the following approaches.

- Conference with school/ Agency Staff
- I.E.P. Review- this may be requested at any time.
- Mediation- A neutral third person assets parents and the school to find a satisfactory solution to their dispute.

- Due Process Hearing- A legal proceeding, it is advise that you obtain legal advice.
- Complaint Resolution Procedure- A complaint that is filed alleging that the local educational agency has not met the requirement of I.D.E.A.. The complaint must be written and signed. The complaint must site the specific I.D.E.A. requirement that was violated and the facts upon which the allegations were made. The state educational agency must resolve the issues within (60) calendar days after the complaint is filed.

IMPORTANT!!

The above mentioned processes may differ in your area. Always check with your local area.

CREDIT:

The proceeding I.E.P. section is an example of the knowledge you need to acquire to become a valued team member in your child's education. I must thank the staff at Baudhuin for providing valuable information to help us maximize Shane's potential.

We also learned specific techniques to help with Shane's progressions and minimize any regressions.

Although Erica Grub introduced us to the benefits of P.E.C.S. (Picture Exchange Communication System) and Miss Nicole showed us a complete system. We were provided with a book of visuals and the skills to properly help Shane throughout his day. These pictures included different foods, drinks, places to go and his favorite toys and activities. The idea was that if he desired something, he would have to remove the Velcro attached picture from the book and bring it to us. This helped to reduce his frustration, by giving him a way to communicate and gave us the ability to increase his verbal skills.

Beside verbal skills, structure is probably the most important tool for a child with autism. Using P.E.C.S. and visuals, we found a way to structure his daily activities. We created a board of visuals that included fun activities as well as daily needs such as bath and bedtime. Just like the book, when it was time to do a certain activity, we would tell him and he would have to bring the picture of the requested activity. Admittedly, we were not as diligent as his teachers, but it seemed to keep him focused.

After several months at Baudhuin, Shane's re-focus periods began to vary in time and intensity. We understood that he was being asked to do more, so this seemed to be in the natural order of the process. Nevertheless, during these times, my stress level would sky rocket, because sometimes life happens and you need to do things and keep appointments.

The best technique and the secret to my sanity on many occasions was a digital egg timer. We were taught this technique in order to place a time limit on his re-focus periods. During a re-focus period, we would put two minutes on the timer, lie it next to him while telling him that he had two minutes to get himself together. After several attempts, Shane began to respond quickly to the timer and I believe he felt that he had some control of his re-focus periods. This technique was so successful, that I began to constantly carry a timer. Today, we rarely need the timer because of this technique, we now can verbally place time limits to re-focus him.

Toward the end of Shane's first year at Baudhuin, we were dealt another challenge. We were losing Miss Nicole as his teacher due to a promotion. Although we were saddened by Miss Nicole leaving the classroom, we were grateful to have Miss Erica Baisley as his new teacher.

Miss Erica had already been working with Shane and displayed an obvious passion for teaching children with special needs. We knew his educational process would remain constant with the potential to expand it. Because she adored Shane and he usually responded well to whatever she asked of him. During his time with Miss Erica, he became more verbal with his requests and social skills. We would get feedback on how he began to greet his classmates and visitors.

But as we discovered, any progressions comes with a regression, unfortunately there always seems to be a trade off.

We were aware of Shane's hypersensitivity to other children's meltdowns, but it was becoming more pronounced. Every time another child would have a meltdown, Shane would cower in a corner and cry. Over the next six to eight months, these episodes were less frequent, due to work and structure provided by Miss Erica and her aides. Another regression, we were introduced to a new twist on his inability to focus. Shane was finding it difficult to complete his tasks (coloring, puzzles, etc.) due to the urge to help his classmates with their tasks. Whether it was boredom or lack of focus, this could present a major problem to his educational process in the future.

Thanks to both Miss Nicole and Miss Erica, we discovered we would be losing Miss Erica for his second year. This time it was because of Shane's promotion. The first year closing I.E.P. illustrated how he met the majority of his goals. We agreed he should be placed in a mid-level class for his second and final year at Baudhuin. The mid level class comprised of ten children covering most of the autism spectrum. Some were higher functioning than Shane, while others were lower functioning. The idea was to put Shane with children he could grow to while the others could grow to him. There was some anxiety with the change but to a much lesser degree, because we developed a great working relationship and trust with Shane's team members.

After one year at Baudhuin and working with their incredible staff, we developed a good intuition for people that work with Shane. The second year looked promising after meeting his new teacher, Miss Erikka Volez. Immediately, she struck me as a kind woman who really cared for her students. Initially, Shane displayed his usual shyness, but soon warmed up to her. He would become her best "helper", if one of Shane's classmates broke ranks with the routine, he was the first say "uh-oh" while pointing out the guilty person. For me it was another trade off, he was still displaying his inability to focus and was easily distracted, yet he was actually beginning to initiate his own actions, another victory. During the year, Shane was becoming more verbal due to the work of Miss Erikka and Miss Caroline Bowman, his Speech Pathologist.

His second year dealt more with his social skills. Once a week, Miss Erikka would integrate the class with some typical children and we usually received positive feedback on Shane's interaction. During the year, he still would have his meltdowns, but overall we saw him grow, socially. Our greatest victory was that he was partially potty trained (pee-pee only). Since he responded so well to the timer, Miss Erikka suggested we use for potty training. Initially, we worked in twenty minute intervals. When the timer sounded, we would take him into the bathroom and hope he had the urge. We would reward him with praise and a toy from a treasure box we created. Every week we would decrease the intervals by five minutes and after a couple of months, we had mastered the daytime hours. The nighttime hours took a few more months, because honestly we did not want to give up diapers in lieu of sleeping through the night.

Although we were ecstatic about Shane's growth, we were saddened about his age, five years old. Unfortunately, Baudhuin only takes Pre-K students between the ages of 3 to 5 years old. We knew we would soon have to leave the "bubble" and enroll Shane into a public school kindergarten.

During the year, I attended several classes regarding this transition, yet we were frighten of what awaited us in his immediate future.

Our final I.E.P. for Shane was to determine what school he would attend and the services he would receive. This meeting would include members of the two potential schools he would attend, as well as the members of Shane's team at Baudhuin. The two schools represented were a General Education with minimal support and the other school would offer him total support in a "cluster" class. A cluster class is comprised of other children with special needs and a teaching staff that specializes with these students. Although we saw tremendous growth in Shane, we felt there was a lot more to be done. After the discussion, we found that all parties agreed on two major points. One, he would benefit from a cluster class and two, that he would benefit from working in general education classroom with support of an aide. The placement ratio we agreed upon was a 50/50 split with an increase to his speech and occupational therapy services. We anticipated more changes and anxiety. We felt it was a good start for Shane and as long as we were involved with his new school and building new relationships with his teachers and the staff.

Shane's graduation day from Baudhuin was a day full of tears and smiles. He walked out with his cap and gown and froze after seeing the roomful of parents. Our proudest moment was a gift that three years prior we could have never imagined receiving. The son who never looked up- looked into and scanned the audience for his mama and dada.

Heartfelt Thanks

I have often looked at the following list of "Shane's Team" in two ways. First, our little man is a child with autism and requires the expertise of these people to reach his maximum potential. And second, in a world that is too often cynical and selfish, we found people who sincerely care for others.

First , I want to thank Nancy, an incredible wife, friend, and mother. She has always been my rock through the rough times and the perfect partner to celebrate the smallest of victories. She gives her heart and soul to Shane and is always consumed with thoughts of what would benefit him. Shane and I are fortunate to have her in our lives. I could not imagine taking this journey with anyone else.

We would like to thank our families, because without them, this would have been a far more difficult journey.

We are fortunate to have Nancy's family so close. They are always eager to spend time with him, whenever we need them. This alone time is so important to us, it gives us time to re-connect with each other. They have shown incredible patience and have been a great influence on him.

We are grateful to my father who lives in Tennessee, for his support and willingness to make the long drive to visit us a few times a year. He has developed a habit that I believe may be useful to others who have distant families that may visit your family. Before each visit, he always asks if Shane has any new quirks and how we handle them. I believe this makes his visit more pleasurable and memorable for both of them. And thank you to my mother for her support.

And to my daughter, Jessica (Sissy), who has been made to endure time lost with us due to his rigid schedule. Thank you for your love of Shane and understanding.

Earlier I mentioned that you need two important tools, support and knowledge. Without a team, support and knowledge would not be possible. Nancy and I realize that the words, thank you could never be enough. We wanted to let them know that their hard work and commitment really do change lives.

Shane's Team

· Ellen Wood, D.O. (Fertility Specialist)

Roberto F. Tucchman, M.D., F.A.A.N., F.A.A.P.: Neurologist

Monica Ventura: Speech Pathologist

Erica Grub: Speech Pathologist

Sherry Swanson: Broward County Schools- Pre K Agency Liaison

Michelle Kaplan: Director of Baudhuin

Carol Cheli: Baudhuin Administrator

Nicole Gaskin-Daniels: Teacher, Baudhuin

Erica Baisley: Teacher, Baudhuin

Erikka Volez: Teacher, Baudhuin

Manny Abreau- Gonzalez, PhD : Support and Education, Baudhuin

Caroline Bowman: Evaluation Specialist, Baudhuin

Belinda Perez: Occupational Therapist, Baudhuin

Jennifer Carr- Hertel: Occupational Therapist, Baudhuin

Karla-Ann Hall: LEA Representative, Baudhuin

Tammy Gipps: Family Counselor, Baudhuin

The parents from Baudhuin for their support and friendship.

The South Florida autism community.

Children's Medical Center: Shane's pediatric group, but most important, a constant source of support and strength.

Autism Speaks (www.autismspeaks.org)

Autism Society of America (www.autism-society.org)

The star of Shane's Team is Shane. He has worked hard and made tremendous progress. They say all children have a gift. Shane's gift is his persistence and that he works hard to please those he feels comfortable with. Shane, if you never spontaneously say I Love You, we still see it your beautiful eyes. Thank you for allowing us to be your parents.

FinalThoughts

If you suspect any delays, seek help, the last thing your child needs is an ostrich. Each day lost keeps your child trapped in their own little world that much longer.

If your child is diagnosed with autism, the natural response is to blame yourself, it was part of my process. But remember, autism affects 1 in every 150 children covering all races, ethnicities, and socioeconomic levels. Do not feel ashamed of your child; be proud. Proud, because every victory they experience will be the results of hard work on their part.

Once diagnosed, you have two responsibilities. One, to become the best advocate for your child in public, in school, and all facets of their lives; including their families. We immediately told our families (which must be a personal choice), for support and to keep consistencies with the structures we have created for him. Another concern must be safety for any family members or professionals who interact with your child. They should be made aware of any possibilities that the child may "bolt" or risk injury with head banging or throwing themselves on the floor. They should be aware of the child's "quirks", whether it is ignoring people and/or inappropriate emotional outbursts. These are the child's "quirks" and must not be taken personally. Second, get educated and stay updated with the constant changes in your rights, autism research, and therapies available. To aide you in this task, seek out your local autism support agency through the school system. Another option would be national organizations such as, Autism Speaks and Autism Society of America.

Most fathers secretly wish that someday their sons hit's a World Series homerun or throws the winning Super Bowl pass. I must admit I was one of those fathers.

Today, my dream for Shane is that he is happy and never loses that persistence that allows him to always raise the bar of his potential.

About the Author

This is Tim's second published book through Authorhouse. In 2005, he published Blood, Sweat-No Fears, Handling Medical Emergencies with Confidence. The book desrcibed the signs and symptoms of medical emergencies through rescue stories and scenarios. In 2006, Tim was fortunate enough to have a story (The Reunion) he submitted included in Tim Russert's, Wisdom of Our Fathers. In the tradition of story telling that Tim has developed, I Love U gives the reader an insight to the signs of autism through stories in thier daily life.